Y0-DDS-239

Contents

3

Introduction

People are taking CBD (cannabidiol) to help relieve pain, improve sleep, and treat anxiety. They are buying CBD capsules, oils, vapes, and edibles to achieve this relief. And while clinical research on the efficacy of CBD across applications is limited, anecdotal evidence is strong.

But it's hard to know what CBD gummies to buy. Especially in the edible category where everything looks tasty. It's also hard to know how much to take, how long they take to work, and what brands are best.

So, let's talk about CBD gummies. In this article we'll explain to you what these edibles are, how to pick the right one for you, and how to get a proper dose. We have to start with the meaning of CBD

CBD

Cannabidiol is a chemical in the Cannabis sativa plant, also known as marijuana or hemp. Over 80 chemicals, known as cannabinoids, have been identified in the Cannabis sativa plant. While delta-9-tetrahydrocannabinol (THC) is the major active ingredient in marijuana, cannabidiol is also obtained from hemp, which contains only very small amounts of THC.

The passage of the 2018 Farm Bill made it legal to sell hemp and hemp products in the U.S. But that doesn't mean that all hemp-derived cannabidiol products are legal. Since cannabidiol has been studied as a new drug, it can't be legally included in foods or dietary supplements. Also, cannabidiol can't be included in products marketed with therapeutic claims. Cannabidiol can only be included in "cosmetic" products and only if it contains less than 0.3% THC. But there are still products labeled as dietary supplements on the market that contain cannabidiol. The amount of cannabidiol contained in these products is not always reported accurately on the product label.

Cannabidiol is most commonly used for seizure disorder (epilepsy). It is also used for anxiety, pain, a muscle disorder called dystonia, Parkinson disease, Crohn disease, and many other conditions, but there is no good scientific evidence to support these uses.

How does it work

Cannabidiol has antipsychotic effects. The exact cause for these effects is not clear. But cannabidiol seems to prevent the breakdown of a chemical in the brain that affects pain, mood, and mental function. Preventing the breakdown of this chemical and increasing its levels in the blood seems to reduce psychotic symptoms associated with conditions such as schizophrenia. Cannabidiol might also block some of the psychoactive effects of delta-9-tetrahydrocannabinol (THC). Also, cannabidiol seems to reduce pain and anxiety.

Uses & Effectiveness

Likely Effective for

Seizure disorder (epilepsy). A specific cannabidiol product (Epidiolex, GW Pharmaceuticals) has been shown to reduce seizures in adults and children with various conditions that are linked with seizures. This product is a prescription drug for treating seizures caused by Dravet syndrome or Lennox-Gastaut syndrome. It has also been shown to reduce seizures in people with tuberous sclerosis complex, Sturge-Weber syndrome, febrile infection-related epilepsy syndrome (FIRES), and specific genetic disorders that cause epileptic encephalopathy. But it's not approved for treating these other types of seizures.

Possibly Effective for

Multiple sclerosis (MS). A prescription-only nasal spray product (Sativex, GW Pharmaceuticals) containing both 9-delta-tetrahydrocannabinol (THC) and cannabidiol has been shown to be effective for improving pain, muscle-tightness, and urination frequency in people with MS. This product is used in over 25 countries outside of the United States. But there is inconsistent evidence on the effectiveness of cannabidiol for symptoms of multiple sclerosis when it is used alone. Some early research suggests that using a cannabidiol spray under the tongue might improve pain and muscle tightness, but not muscle spasms, tiredness, bladder control, mobility, or well-being and quality of life in patients with MS.

Insufficient Evidence for

- Bipolar disorder. Early reports show that taking cannabidiol does not improve manic episodes in people with bipolar disorders.

- A type of inflammatory bowel disease (Crohn disease). Early research shows that taking cannabidioldoes not reduce disease activity in adults with Crohn disease.

- Diabetes. Early research shows that taking cannabidiol does not improve blood glucose levels, blood insulin levels, or HbA1c in adults with type 2 diabetes.

- A movement disorder marked by involuntary muscle contractions (dystonia). Early research suggests that taking cannabidiol daily for 6 weeks might improve dystonia by 20% to 50% in some people. Higher quality research is needed to confirm this.

- A condition in which a transplant attacks the body (graft-versus-host disease or GVHD). Graft-versus-host disease is a complication that can occur after a bone marrow transplant. In people with this condition, donor cells attack the person's own cells. Early research shows that taking cannabidiol daily starting 7 days before bone marrow transplant and continuing for 30 days after transplant can extend the time it takes for a person to develop GVHD.

- An inherited brain disorder that affects movements, emotions, and thinking (Huntington disease). Early research shows that taking cannabidiol daily does not improve symptoms of Huntington's disease.

- Insomnia. Early research suggests that taking 160 mg of cannabidiol before bed improves sleep time in people with insomnia. However, lower doses do not have this effect. Cannabidiol also does not seem to help people fall asleep and might reduce the ability to recall dreams.
- Multiple sclerosis (MS). There is inconsistent evidence on the effectiveness of cannabidiol for symptoms of multiple sclerosis. Some early

research suggests that using a cannabidiol spray under the tongue might improve pain and muscle tightness in people with MS. However, it does not appear to improve muscle spasms, tiredness, bladder control, the ability to move around, or well-being and quality of life.

- Withdrawal from heroin, morphine, and other opioid drugs. Early research shows that taking cannabidiol for 3 days reduces cravings and anxiety in people with heroin use disorder that are not using heroin or any other opioid drugs.

- Parkinson disease. Some early research shows that taking cannabidiol daily for 4 weeks improves psychotic symptoms in people with Parkinson disease and psychosis.

- Schizophrenia. Research on the use of cannabidiol for psychotic symptoms in people with schizophrenia is conflicting. Some early research suggests that taking cannabidiol four times daily for 4 weeks improves psychotic symptoms and might be as effective as the antipsychotic medication amisulpride. However, other early research suggests that taking cannabidiol for 14 days is not beneficial. The conflicting results might be related to the cannabidiol dose used and duration of treatment.

- Quitting smoking. Early research suggests that inhaling cannabidiol with an inhaler for one week might reduce the number of cigarettes smoked by about 40% compared to baseline.

A type of anxiety marked by fear in some or all social settings (social anxiety disorder). Some early research shows that taking cannabidiol 300 mg daily does not improve anxiety during public speaking in people with social anxiety disorder. However, other early research in people with social anxiety disorder suggests that taking a higher dose (400-600 mg) may improve anxiety associated with public speaking or medical imaging testing. Also, some research in people who do not have social anxiety disorder shows that taking cannabidiol 300 mg might reduce anxiety during public speaking.

Side Effects & Safety

When taken by mouth: Cannabidiol is POSSIBLY SAFE when taken by mouth or sprayed under the tongue appropriately. Cannabidiol in doses of up to 300 mg daily have been taken by mouth safely for up to 6 months. Higher doses of 1200-1500 mg daily have been taken by mouth safely for up to 4 weeks. A prescription cannabidiol product (Epidiolex) is approved to be taken by mouth in doses of up to 10-20 mg/kg daily. Cannabidiol sprays that are applied under the tongue have been used in doses of 2.5 mg for up to 2 weeks.

Some reported side effects of cannabidiol include dry mouth, low blood pressure, light headedness, and drowsiness. Signs of liver injury have also been reported in some patients, but this is less common.

When applied to the skin: There isn't enough reliable information to know if cannabidiol is safe or what the side effects might be.

Special Precautions & Warnings

- Pregnancy and breast-feeding: There is not enough reliable information about the safety of taking cannabidiol if you are pregnant or breast feeding. Stay on the safe side and avoid use.

- Children: A prescription cannabidiol product (Epidiolex) is POSSIBLY SAFE when taken by mouth daily. The most common dose used is 10 mg/kg daily. Higher doses of 15-20 mg/kg daily may be used in some children, but these higher doses are more likely to cause side effects. This product is approved for use in certain children 2 years of age and older, but has been used in children as young as 1 year of age.

- Parkinson disease: Some early research suggests that taking high doses of cannabidiol might make muscle movement and tremors worse in people with Parkinson disease.

The difference between Cannabis and Industrial Hemp

To understand the legal status of hemp and cannabis and products derived from them we must first know the difference between hemp and cannabis itself and CBD-based products, Hemp-based products and Cannabis derived products:

- Cannabis or Cannabis Sativa – is a plant indigenous to and originating from Central and upper South Asia. Three species are recognized: Cannabis sativa, Cannabis indica, and Cannabis ruderalis although due to constant natural and human-based cross-breeding of species, they rarely appear in their original form. Total THC levels in today's Cannabis Sativa strains are usually very high – up to 30%.

- Hemp, or industrial hemp – are registered strains of the Cannabis Sativa plant subspecies that are grown for a variety of industrial and commercial uses. Hemp can be used for extraction of cannabinoids and can be refined into a variety of commercial products that don't contain cannabinoids. Total THC levels in industrial hemp are usually very low – up to 1%

- CBD-based products – are products that contain different concentrations of CBD or Cannabidiol – a non-psychoactive cannabinoid present in all Cannabis Sativa strains including Hemp. We must underline that the CBD used can be of full spectrum or crystals(Isolate).

- Full spectrum CBD (along with other 140+ cannabinoids) is usually extracted from registered Hemp strains but can be also extracted from all other subspecies of Cannabis Sativa. In order to maintain the THC concentrations below the legally allowed limits, the extract is usually further elaborated. CBD Crystals or CBD Isolate begins as hemp-derived CBD extract. Then, all other plants natural cannabinoids and other compounds except for CBD are removed, leaving CBD as a pure crystalline, making CBD legal for sales also in countries where THC concentration is limited to 0.0%.

- Hemp-based products – are products made from industrial hemp and do not contain cannabinoids. With the reintroduction of hemp in western society – industries we can observe a boom of new hemp-based products such as paper, textiles, clothing, biodegradable plastics, animal feed, insulation, construction material, biofuel, food...

- Cannabis-derived products – are products made from Cannabis Sativa and Cannabis Sativa plant parts usually containing elevated concentrations of THC.

Our CBD map helps our user to quickly identify the legality of CBD products in different countries. It can be helpful when you need in-depth information about the CBD law and regulations regarding also the legal status of THC and its allowed limit in hemp and CBD-based products. You can access this information by simply clicking on a pin marked on the country map. We strongly advise you to do detailed research on the latest laws and regulations regarding CBD and THC before travelling to another country and we wouldn't advise you to bring any CBD based products on a plane, even if the THC content is below 0,2%. Instead, we advise you to order beforehand your preferred CBD products to your designated location.

CBD GUMMIES

CBD gummies are starting to become very popular as a daily supplement. They are gaining a lot of popularity among families that want to enjoy the full benefits of cannabidiol in a form that's easy to swallow. When CBD is in gummy form, it makes it much easier and much more enjoyable for kids and pets to consume. Adults enjoy taking them as a daily treat too. Just like regular gummies, CBD gummies are available in fun shapes like little rainbow teddy bears, and both sweet and sour flavors. For those not used to CBD, it helps to know what exactly CBD Gummies are and what they do. CBD comes in many forms, from tincture oils to topical cream products. Gummies are a form of CBD edible. In other words, all you need to do is eat these tasty treats to get the effects of CBD.

CBD Gummies taste like your favorite sweets. You can get them as sweet fruit gums, gummy bears or even sour gummies. These make for a fun and easy way to get all the effects of CBD.

While your doctor might recommend you go easy on the sweets, these are packed with health benefits. CBD helps you relieve pain, reduce stress and anxiety, and prevent a range of illnesses. It also has antibacterial, antioxidant, antipsychotic, and even anticancer effects. It's used for various conditions, from Arthritis to epilepsy. CBD Gummies are a fantastic health product for those who want its impressive medical perks.

Where To Buy CBD Gummies

It's easier than ever to get your hands on CBD Gummies in a safe and legal manner. While cannabis is still banned in many parts of the states, hemp-derived CBD products are legal across the country. That means you can buy these with no limits on age and possession.

The best way to get them is to buy CBD Gummies online. JustCBDStore offers a range of CBD Gummies that can whet anyone's appetite and treat their medical needs. These are all made with hemp CBD Oil so you can legally order them for delivery and use them anywhere in the US.

There are various CBD Gummies to choose from. For instance, you might like clear gummy bears or you may prefer sour worms. These mimic your favorite treats, only they're full of the medical goodness of CBD. You can also get them in higher quantities. For instance, the CBD Gummies Party Pack will give you 3000mg of assorted CBD Gummies to last you for a long time.

Why Use CBD Gummies

There are plenty of options when it comes to using CBD. For instance, some users may enjoy the simplicity of CBD Tincture while others may prefer the experience of vaping CBD. However, CBD Gummies have a few benefits which make them a preferred product for many.

Of course, one of the main reasons to take CBD Gummies is that they taste good. Users can enjoy these as a snack while also getting the wide-ranging benefits of CBD. Who doesn't want to enjoy their favorite candies and still improve their health while eating them?

CBD Gummies are also very useful for controlling your CBD dosage. These are split into small serving sizes of around 10-25mg of CBD. So, for instance, those who need a 100mg daily dose can eat 10 a day to make sure they get what they need. You can buy gummies in various quantities, so no matter how much CBD you need, it's easy to get your daily dosage.

They also make using CBD simple. While not everyone is used to vaping or sublingually taking oil, everyone can enjoy eating gummy sweets without any hassle. They're suitable for any age and can treat all kinds of medical conditions and health issues.

How Many CBD Gummies to Take

The amount of CBD Gummies you should consume depends on a few factors. Your recommended CBD dosage varies depending on what you're using it for. For instance, those who need general health effects might only want a 10-25mg daily dose. Those who need to treat seizures or anxiety may need up to 600mg of CBD.

The severity of your symptoms can also make a difference. Those who want to relieve severe anxiety symptoms might want to take a high dosage to relieve the problem fast. However, those with mild symptoms may benefit more from a smaller day-by-day dosage which will take effect over time.

Your bodyweight can also make a difference. Smaller and lighter users will need less CBD than a larger, heavier user. With CBD Gummies, your metabolism may also make a difference. Those with fast metabolisms will digest and get the effects of CBD faster.

Taking 10-25mg of CBD a day is a good starting point. This dosage can help you get the general health effects of CBD such as less stress and prevention of illness. However, those who need to treat specific symptoms or conditions will have different recommended dosages.

Dosages

CBD Gummies are one of the best ways to get your daily dose of CBD. Not only do they offer an incredibly simple way to get the right amount of CBD, but they also taste great. These CBD edibles are split into small serving sizes of 10-25mg of CBD, making it incredibly easy to get the amount you need for whatever you're trying to treat.

CBD dosages can be confusing for some. Different ailments require different amounts of CBD. The best dosage for you can also depend on your body size and the severity of your symptoms. The good news is that you can't overdose or get ill from too much CBD, so you can take as much as you want. However, you'll still want to make sure you're not wasting any.

So how many CBD Gummies do you need? It really depends on what you need them for. Those who want general health benefits will need far less than someone treating chronic pain, for instance. But there is a lot of research to let us know the best CBD dosages. Here's a CBD Gummies dosage guide to help

CBD Gummies Dosage for Pain

Pain is one of the most common symptoms people treat with CBD. Studies show that CBD can help with severe chronic pain as well as general strains, aches, and physical discomfort. It binds to cannabinoid receptors in the body and brain to reduce inflammation, speed up the healing process, and even lessen the sensation of pain.

Studies suggest that taking 15-25mg of CBD daily is helpful for pain. This makes it simple to manage pain with CBD Gummies. For instance, a 500mg jar of CBD Gummies can last for over a month if you only need a small amount. These are split into servings of either 10mg, 14mg or 25mg, so no matter how much you need, you can easily get the right dosage.

The best dosage for you can depend on your symptoms. For instance, those with severe pain may benefit from even higher dosages. CBD is safe to use in any amount, so if you aren't getting pain relief from a smaller dosage, take an extra gummy to see if it helps.

CBD Gummies Dosage for Anxiety

Anxiety is another issue which people generally use CBD to deal with. Various studies show that CBD can help reduce symptoms of anxiety and help with numerous disorders. It's effective for treating generalized anxiety disorder, social anxiety, PTSD, OCD, and other forms of anxiety.

Research suggests that a higher dosage of CBD is best for numbing anxiety symptoms. For instance, a study found that a single dose of 600mg of CBD helped reduce social anxiety. Other studies found that anywhere from 100mg-600mg of CBD will reduce anxiety.

Again, this can depend on the nature and severity of your symptoms. However, it seems that higher dosages work best for anxiety patients. Luckily, you can buy CBD Gummies in jars of 1000mg or even 3000mg. While they're split into small servings, you can snack on these to get the exact dosage you need.

CBD Gummies Dosage for Seizures

Epilepsy patients also often use CBD to treat seizures. While some forms of epilepsy are hard to treat, research shows that taking CBD regularly can help reduce seizures and may even eliminate them in some patients. Generally, this requires high dosages of CBD.

Seizure dosages are usually based on body weight. Research suggests that around 25mg of CBD per kg of body weight can help reduce seizures. A clinical trial on using CBD for Dravet syndrome found that a dosage of 20mg per kg of body weight was ideal for reducing seizures in patients.

However, taking such a high dosage can be costly and inefficient. Other studies suggest that around 200-300mg of CBD per day can help epileptic patients. While oil is usually used, those who want to medicate with CBD Gummies are best served by a 3000mg jar.

CBD Gummies Dosage for Sleep

CBD also has benefits for sleep. In higher dosages, CBD has sedative effects, which can help users with insomnia. In lower dosages, it can still provide some effects, such as reduced dream recall and increased alertness in the morning. Research shows that CBD helps with REM sleep behavior disorder and daytime fatigue.

As for the right dosage, one study tested doses of 40, 80, and 160mg of CBD. It found that 160mg of CBD was ideal for treating insomnia and helping patients get more sleep. 40 and 80mg still had effects, such as reducing dream recall to help those with recurring nightmares.

This suggests that a high dosage of 160mg may help those with insomnia treat symptoms quickly. However, taking a small daily dosage over time can also help over time. Since CBD Gummies come in 10mg servings, it's easy to control how much you want to either get a small or larger dosage. You can even experiment with both and see what works for you.

CBD Gummies Dosage for Depression

CBD can also help users tackle depression. It has a range of positive effects on your mental health, which includes reducing the symptoms of depression. Additionally, it can help with related issues, such as anxiety and chronic stress.

A 2018 study found that a single dosage of 7-30mg of CBD per kg of body weight rapidly reduced depression. Not only did it help treat depression within 30 minutes, but the positive effects remained for a week. While this study was done on rats, it has promising implications for humans.

Much like with anxiety, a high dose may be ideal for tackling symptoms instantly. A single 400-600mg dose of CBD may be enough to instantly treat symptoms of depression. Users can also take a smaller amount over time for sustained effects. A 3000mg jar of CBD Gummies can give you all the CBD you need for this purpose.

CBD Gummies for Anxiety and Depression

For those of us dealing with anxiety and depression, CBD edibles may hold the key to less worrying, better sleep, and an overall improved quality of life. But out of all the products that exist on the market, CBD gummies are probably the most popular edibles.

The CBD oil used to produce these edibles is extracted from carefully-selected types of cannabis, with low THC and a high concentration of cannabidiol. CBD-based products are part of a different category of medicinal marijuana, one that does not place emphasis on the psychoactive effects of the plant, but rather the curative properties of marijuana.As we mentioned before, the main reason why CBD products have gained such massive popularity is that they offer a natural alternative to medication and other treatment options that carry a certain amount of risk.According to recent studies, cannabidiol is a potentially viable treatment option for anxiety disorders can regulate emotions and emotional memory processing and may also prove useful in solving the current opioid epidemic. If we are to ask the countless individuals who've used cannabidiol, in the form of CBD gummies, oils, balms, and all sorts of edibles, most of them would say this compound has helped them relax, sleep better, manage stress, and improve their overall quality of life.Since the 'CBD boom' has only recently taken the world by surprise, imagine what exciting discoveries researchers might uncover in the coming years.

Throughout our lives, each of us has probably faced the unpleasant symptoms associated with anxiety at least a couple of time. The constant worrying; the sleepless nights; the inability to get a handle on our anxious thoughts.

But when anxiety becomes a constant part of our lives, things can get quite overwhelming. When you can't even muster the courage to get out of the house, you risk losing your job, which in turn gives rise to even more problems.

Fortunately, products such as CBD gummies and other edibles can have a significantly positive impact on anxiety. In fact, numerous anxiety sufferers have reported fewer anxious thoughts, better quality sleep, and a notable improvement in overall mood as a result of using various CBD-based products.

From oils and tinctures to gummies and other edibles, there's an option for every taste, and all of them seem to have the same positive Affecting nearly 322 million people worldwide, depression has recently become the #1 cause of disability. This mood disorder can turn your entire life upside down, causing emotional pain, low self-esteem, fatigue, sleep-related problems, feelings of helplessness, and even thoughts of suicide.

Although researchers and mental health professionals have spent decades studying this condition, there are times when 'traditional' treatments don't seem to work. Affecting nearly 322 million people worldwide, depression has recently become the #1 cause of disability. This mood disorder can turn your entire life upside down, causing emotional pain, low self-esteem, fatigue, sleep-related problems, feelings of helplessness, and even thoughts of suicide.

Although researchers and mental health professionals have spent decades studying this condition, there are times when 'traditional' treatments don't seem to work.Since therapy takes time and medication has numerous unpleasant side effects, perhaps a good alternative would be CBD-based products.Many depression sufferers have discovered that this natural option proves to be quite useful in alleviating the troublesome effects of depression. By interacting with the endocannabinoid system, edibles like CBD gummies prove to be highly effective in regulating mood, sleep, appetite, and even pain.

Research into CBD is still relatively new, so most long-term studies are currently in-progress. However there is some developing research about CBD's impact on anxiety and depression that shows this botanical compound has the power to do more than chill you out.

If you have certain medical issues that you feel could be effectively treated with CBD, you should speak to your doctor. Ultimately, our full spectrum CBD products are formulated in an attempt to decrease the strain you feel mentally, emotionally, and physically day-to-day. However your doctor may have a different opinion and suggest an alternative to taking CBD.

What If Your CBD Dosage Doesn't Work

While studies shine some light on CBD dosages that might work, it can still vary. Some users may only need a moderate amount of CBD, while some might find they need more. However, it's safe to increase your dosage of CBD if you find your symptoms aren't treated.

CBD Gummies enable you to increase your dosage by a small amount each time. Since they come with around 10-25mg of CBD per gummy, you can easily take one more per day to see if it works better for you.

It can also help to discuss your condition with a doctor. They may be able to help with recommended dosages or additional treatments to help your symptoms. In addition to the problems listed above, CBD can also help with things like schizophrenia, neurological disorders, addiction, skin problems, and more.

However, don't worry about taking too much CBD. Research regularly shows that it's a safe treatment with no harmful long-term effects. What's more, you can't overdose on CBD or get addicted. This makes it a safe and effective alternative to other treatments which may cause negative side effects or result in dependence.

HEALTH BENEFITS OF CBD GUMMIES

Many of us loved eating gummy bears as kids, but did you know there are now gummies with healing benefits?Alongside the thousands of people enjoying the benefits of CBD oil as a tincture, CBD gummies are quickly increasing in popularity. These delicious candies offer the same benefits as other forms of CBD, but many people enjoy taking them in this form for a variety of reasons, including their great flavor.Cannabidiol, also known as CBD is one of many naturally occurring chemicals found in cannabis. Unlike THC, which is CBD's better known cousin and the main active ingredient in psychoactive cannabis, CBD doesn't get you "high." Instead, CBD users report it benefits a host of ailments, from chronic pain to schizophrenia. It's even been shown to benefit kids with epilepsy.People seek out CBD because it has few side effects compared to its numerous potential benefits. And, fortunately, CBD is widely available to consumers in all 50 states. In this article, we look at why CBD gummies are becoming a preferred nutritional supplement for so many.

CBD EDIBLES

It is important to always read the label to know exactly what you are buying and consuming but you can rest assured that CBD gummies from reputable brands are organic (unless stated otherwise). These gummies are made of natural ingredients and are then infused with organic CBD. As the result, you get an amazing tasting and HEALTHY CBD Gummy. There are no harmful chemicals or stimulants either.

SCIENCE ON CBD FOR PAIN, INSOMNIA, INFLAMMATION AND ANXIETY

A growing body of evidence on cannabidiol has shown through multiple studies and medical tests that it aids in alleviating pain of many kinds. Some CBD users have stopped taking over the counter drugs or pharmaceuticals because CBD helps them so much. Studies of CBD also show it could help people with sleep, inflammation, and anxiety.

- CHRONIC PAIN: "Specifically, cannabis extracts (THC & CBD) have shown effectiveness to relief some symptoms of the patients with multiple sclerosis, mainly for pain and spasticity."

- Insomnia and sleep disorders: "The systemic acute administration of CBD appears to increase total sleep time, in addition to increasing sleep latency in the light period of the day of administration."

- Inflammation: "Specifically, cannabis extracts (THC & CBD) have shown effectiveness to relief some symptoms of the patients with multiple sclerosis, mainly for pain and spasticity."

- Anxiety: "Studies using animal models of anxiety and involving healthy volunteers clearly suggest an anxiolytic-like effect of CBD. Moreover, CBD was shown to reduce anxiety in patients with social anxiety disorder."

CBD GUMMIES VS THC GUMMIES

In states where psychoactive cannabis (marijuana) is legal for recreational or medicinal purposes, THC gummies are also available. What differentiates these two products is whether they contain Cannabidiol (CBD) or Tetrahydrocannabinol (THC).

However, while THC is psychoactive (it gets you "high"), CBD is not. While many people prefer CBD because they find it doesn't interfere as much with their daily lives, nonetheless THC has many benefits, especially as a pain killer. Nonetheless, both options provide many potential healing benefits and we hope all forms of cannabis will someday be available legally throughout the United States. In the meantime, be sure to obey your local laws.

While you can effectively take CBD as a tincture, swallow it in a capsule, or even vape it, CBD is appearing in many new forms, from chocolate to cocktails. We expect that even more innovative and quality CBD brands to appear in the future.It's no surprise, then, that gummies are still best sellers. Whether you are suffering from pain, stress, inflammation, anxiety, depression, or poor sleep … CBD gummies provide a fun and effective way to consume this beneficial cannabinoid.

OTHER BENEFITS CBD GUMMIES OFFER

Millions of people around the world have already benefited from the use of cannabidiol (also known as CBD). Studies reveal it has been used to treat a wide range of issues.Our CBD Gummies don't contain THC and are made from natural ingredients including coconut oil, citric acid, and natural colors and flavors. Our CBD is also grown with clean practices and is pesticide- free, sourced directly from American farms to ensure you can feel confident and healthy in your choice.

Finally, our product is also made without yeast, gluten, dairy, milk, soy, eggs, tree nuts, peanuts, shellfish or fish making it a great choice for most people regardless of dietary concerns or allergens. Please note, due to our use of gelatin, this version of our CBD Gummies are not vegan. You can check out our Vegan AF CBD Gummies product if you need a tasty vegan-friendly solution

WHAT MAKES YOUR CBD GUMMIES DIFFERENT

Unlike some of our competitors which get a lot of their CBD from China and other sources with loose regulatory requirements, our CBD is sourced directly from farms in the USA and grown in accordance with the 2018 Farm Bill. These farms are regulated by the states' Agriculture Departments. This requires our CBD to be pesticide free.And let's be real. We're funny. And that's in our CBD too. Now that is a wellness hack.

HOW CBD GUMMIES WORK

Each one of us has an Endocannabinoid System inside or body, or what we like to call an ECS. The ECS is key in regulating our mood and really how we feel in our body every single day. This system has two receptors: CB1 and CB2. CB2 receptors are found mostly in the immune system, and can reduce inflammation and certain kinds of pain. Research shows that CB2 may be affected in a positive way by cannabinoid type substances, like CBD.

INGREDIENTS & USAGE OF CBD GUMMIES

We keep it real and life and with our ingredients. Everything is sourced here in the USA. And we never add anything in as filler. Every ingredient has a purpose and a place.

FULL SPECTRUM CBD OIL

Absolutely no THC, ever,Vitamin B13 May regulate your nervous system,Vitamin D3,Can boost your immune system,Coconut Oil,Known to provide quick energy, Pure Cane Sugar, Natural sweetness that's just right.

How to use our CBD Gummies

Take 1-3 gummies, a couple of deep breaths and within 20-30 minutes you'll already start to feel your Sunday Scaries melt away. Many of our customers report they feel the effects of our CBD quickly. With that being said it can takes more than one use to really feel the continued chill. Typically it takes 5-7 days for it to build up in your system and be effective. If you have any health conditions or are using any medication please consult with your doctor first.

Will there be any negative side effects of CBD gummies

As with any natural or supplement product, there are always risks associated with consumption. Some of our customers have reported slight dizziness or drowsiness. While we cannot promise that taking our CBD is risk free, we de believe that the chance of being exposed to any major risks are low.

If there are any concerns at all with taking our CBD Gummies then it is worth consulting with a doctor, who can advise further.

Choosing CBD gummies over other forms

Everyone is different, but there are distinct benefits offered by our CBD Gummies. First, our products use the highest quality full-spectrum CBD, which leads to the best possible absorption. They are a portable, convenient option that can easily be taken with you to work, school or anywhere else where you might need a boost. On top of this, it is far more socially acceptable to pop a couple gummies in your mouth in certain social situations than it is to say, pull out a vape pen. Finally, our gummies are vitamin-infused, healthy and, most importantly, tasty!

While other manufacturers of CBD products often use low-quality products shipped from China and other locations with loose, substandard regulations, our focus is on quality, American- owned sources. All our CBD is derived from American farms that grow in accordance with the 2018 Farm Bill. If you are interested in other forms of products you can try our CBD Candy called Unicorn Jerky.

Using CBD gummies for other medical problems

As reported in Medical News Today, CBD has reportedly been used for a solution to life's everyday struggles.

If you have certain medical issues that you feel could be effectively treated with CBD, you should speak to your doctor. Ultimately, our products are formulated to support a happy lifestyle, and your doctor might suggest a different dosage or method of taking CBD. Our products are not intended to diagnose, cure or prevent any disease, and you should speak to a doctor about medication options available.

Are CBD gummies dangerous or unhealthy

Our CBD Gummies are lab tested and include vitamin B12 and Vitamin D3. While most customers find our gummies extremely helpful, if you have concerns over taking CBD, we encourage you to speak with your doctor.

If this is your first time using our CBD Gummies, you might want to start with a single bottle to gauge your body's response to it. Most customers who purchase a single bottle of our CBD Gummies, quickly sign up to become a subscriber.

Subscriptions offer discounts starting at 13% off retail and will ensure you never run out of CBD gummy bears. When you are already struggling with a serious case of the Sunday Scaries, nothing feels worse than realizing you've just hit the end of your bottle of CBD gummies— so a subscription is an ideal way to avoid this.

How do I use CBD tummies

It couldn't be easier. If you have ever eaten a gummy sweet, you will know exactly what to do. You have the option to chew them or suck on them and savor the flavors. As you consume this form of CBD orally, it travels through your digestive system and is absorbed into the gut and bloodstream. As these are edible supplements, they can take a little longer to work, so be patient! As there is 25mg of CBD in each gummy, it is advisable, to begin with half a gummy to see how you react. From there, you can increase or decrease the amount as needed.

How often to take CBD gummies

This, too, can be completely up to you and your own individual needs and preferences. For some users, our CBD Gummies are used on an as-needed basis for when upcoming mid- term exams, high-stakes pitch meetings or just a typical Saturday night leaves you feeling particularly high strung.

For others, CBD is taken frequently or daily. The first step to figuring out your CBD dosage and the frequency you need to take it is to get started with a small dosage and see how you feel. Most customers start with 1-2 CBD gummies, then go from there

Getting addicted to CBD gummies

There are not sufficient studies readily available to answer this question. Whether or not certain substances can be classified as physically addictive depends on several factors, including how it causes human nerve cells to send and receive messages. CBD can promote serotonin reabsorption—something key for those struggling with personal darkness—but it ultimately does not target or interfere with your dopamine production, something that is key to classifying a substance as physically addictive. When you use an addictive substance, your brain's reward system will trick itself into thinking it needs more of said substance to produce any dopamine, a hormone in your brain associated with happiness and rewards.

If you have concerns about becoming addicted to our CBD Gummies, we encourage you to speak with your doctor or trained medical professional.

The mayhem of Sunday Scaries don't have to get the best of you—there are holistic, natural options available that can help like CBD.

Whether you have a heavy exam season, a thousand office deadlines or a classic case of the Sunday Scaries, life can get in the way of your performance and negatively impact your personal and professional life.

In the United States alone, there are 40 million people from all walks of life who are suffering from anxiety. However, many people are wary of the options available to help them. For this reason, many are still searching for stress solutions that are affordable, all-natural, and healthy.

CBD is a cannabinoid derived from hemp that has been used around the world to address several public health concerns, including mood and you can now get it in a delicious CBD gummy bear form.

Here at Sunday Scaries, we know the potential that CBD has on the lives of those living with life's social burdens.

Many of our customers believe our CBD Gummies provide relief without the high of traditional THC products.

UNDERSTAND YOUR LEGAL OBLIGATIONS

Just because the 2018 Farm Bill federally legalized industrial hemp and, by extension, hemp extract, like CBD oils, doesn't mean there aren't significant regulatory considerations surrounding the industrial hemp industry. The 2018 Farm Bill essentially removed CBD from the federal Controlled Substances Act and the oversight of the Drug Enforcement Agency. Instead, it placed governance of the hemp industry and CBD oil in the hands of the Food and Drug Administration (FDA).

Currently, the FDA is still devising regulations, leaving the CBD industry in a sort of gray area. So far, the federal agency has signaled that marketing CBD as having health benefits will not be tolerated. It has also initiated a crackdown against CBD infused foods and beverages in some instances.

Further complicating the regulatory landscape is the 2017 approval of the CBD-based pharmaceutical Epidolex, an epilepsy medication that was approved by the FDA. Since CBD is a main ingredient in an FDA-approved drug, using it in food products without FDA approval could be illegal. Clearer guidance is sorely needed for CBD businesses to operate in compliance with federal regulations.

"I think the FDA does have to step in, and they will," said Slovik. "I expect a lot of changes to labels; we're seeing a lot of businesses out there now using the term 'hemp extract' instead of CBD, or they're not thinking of health benefits so much. Many companies are doing different things, but no one really knows [what the regulations will be] until it happens."Understanding your legal obligations and playing it safe is key in a highly scrutinized industry. While CBD businesses everywhere await clearer regulatory guidance, it is important not to craft your marketing strategy around the supposed benefits of CBD. It's also important to stay apprised of new developments as the FDA moves forward on crafting new regulations.

REASON CBD GUMMY NOT WORKING FOR YOU

- Dosage and tolerance
- Time
- Forms
- It's not for you

Cannabidiol, or CBD, is a nonpsychoactive component found in the Cannabis sativa plant. It's being researched for many possible medical benefits, and unlike tetrahydrocannabinol (THC), this active compound doesn't get you "high."

People are using it to help manage a number of ailments, including:

- chronic pain
- inflammation
- anxiety
- insomnia
- seizures

Before treating a medical condition, speak to your doctor to determine whether CBD is the right option for you, especially if you're taking other medications.

You may have heard some folks with chronic conditions raving about good results — and that's because for them, it's one of the only few options that works.

That said, there are also some legitimate reasons why CBD might not be working for you.

So before you give up on it and tell your CBD-obsessed friends that they're full of it, check to see if any of the following reasons apply to you.

WHERE DID YOU BUY YOUR CBD OIL

As it grows in popularity, it seems like CBD is popping up everywhere from online companies to over-the-counter shops. You might have even tried a free sample to see if it works without investing anything more than the cost of shipping.

Unfortunately, some of these products don't have high-quality CBD. The Food and Drug Administration (FDA) doesn't regulate the industry, and some scammers take full advantage of that fact by selling low-quality products that aren't as potentTrusted Source as they claim to be.

Some have even been found to contain no CBD at all.

So the next time you're looking to invest in a new CBD product, use these three tips to make sure the product lives up to its promises:

Look for evidence of third-party lab tests. Lab testing can reveal exactly how much CBD is in the product, and the test results should be available for you to see for yourself.

Read consumer reviews. Websites like CannaInsider, Leafly, and CBD Oil Users provide reviews on brand effectiveness, delivery time, and customer service.

Pick from a list of well-established brands. Read enough lists of favorite CBD products and you'll see some of the same companies pop up over and over again. Popular brands such as Charlotte's Web, Lazarus Naturals, and CBDistillery have firmly established themselves as quality sources. You can also pick a brand from a list like this one and you won't have to worry about the guesswork of figuring out if the brand you're buying is trustworthy.

Many CBD users have reported trying several different brands before settling on one that works for them, so keep searching if your first try doesn't produce the results you're looking for.

You need to build it up in your system

Finding the right dosage of CBD can be a tricky endeavor. The appropriate amount varies for each individual, as every person has a unique biology that results in a different reaction.

CBD gummies have gained enormous popularity in recent years and it's not hard to see why. Gummies provide a distinctive experience that sets them apart from other forms of CBD. They're not only a fun and convenient way to experience all of the benefits of CBD, but delicious and easy to eat. Here at JustCBD, we mix our top of the line hemp with an extensive amount of appetizing and exciting flavors: so you get all of the same benefits without sacrificing any of the taste. Especially if you are trying CBD for the first time, our CBD gummies are completely safe, convenient, and effective.

Ready for a tasty treat that gives you a real bang for your buck? JustCBD gummy products range from 8mg to 25mg per gummy and are designed with you and your taste buds in mind – so whether you're looking to relieve some stress after a hectic day at the office, or as a delicious bedtime snack to help you drift off to sleep, we have exactly what you're looking for in various sizes and flavors.

CBD Gummy Flavors & Sizes

Many complain about a strong aftertaste with CBD gummies – but that's not a problem for us. Flavor is what we do best. At JustCBD we appreciate everyone has different tastes and we're ready to cater to what you're craving. Our array of flavors include clear bear, sour bear, clear worms, sour worms, happy face, apple rings, peach rings, and blueberry rings. Each flavor is available in different size jars from 250mg, 500mg, 750mg, 1000mg, 3000mg jars.

Cannabidiol, or CBD oil, is a cannabinoid, or naturally occurring biochemical found in cannabis plants. Cannabinoids interact with the endocannabinoid system in humans, and these reactions can affect sleep, mood, pain, and appetite. However, CBD does not produce any psychoactive effects on its own and will not make people feel high, as is the case with other cannabinoids like tetrahydrocannabinol (THC). As a result, CBD oil products are widely used to alleviate symptoms for a wide range of medical conditions and disorders.

CBD oil products come in several different forms. Many users prefer gummy edibles, or gummies, which are ingested orally. Most gummies contain between 5mg and 30mg of CBD, resulting in a mellow interaction that will not cause excessive drowsiness. Many users prefer to take more than one gummy at a time, but optimal dosage depends on the individual's tolerance, as well as age, weight, and other factors.

The CBD oil in most gummies is extracted from hemp plants and has been isolated from THC and other cannabinoids that induce high feelings. These gummies are legal in all 50 states. However, some gummies may contain CBD with trace amounts of THC; the legality of these products varies by state. For this guide, we will focus exclusively on non-THC gummies.

Shopping for the Best CBD Gummies
Many people who use CBD oil prefer to ingest the substance orally in the form of an edible or capsule.

Gummies are one of the most popular edible options for CBD consumers.

Often times, gummies are flavored with fruit juice and other natural ingredients, giving them a distinct, pleasant taste that masks the taste of CBD (which some find bitter and unpleasant). Gummies are also soft and easy to chew, making them a good option for people with dentures or other dental issues who are not well-suited for harder capsules.

Gummies come in a wide range of concentrations, from low-dose 1mg to 10mg options to high-dose gummies of up to 100mg per serving.

Cannabidiol, or CBD, is a cannabinoid found in cannabis plants. Cannabinoids are natural compounds that, when introduced to the human body, react with a communication center known as the endocannabinoid system. These interactions have an effect on functions like appetite, sleep, pain, and mood. As a result, products containing CBD can alleviate symptoms associated with the following conditions:

- Insomnia, other sleep disorders, and general difficulty falling and staying asleep
- Anxiety and stress
- Chronic pain
- Epilepsy
- Cancer, HIV, and other diseases that affect the immune system
- Nausea

Many associate cannabis with marijuana and getting high. However, CBD is different from other tetrahydrocannabinol (THC) and other cannabinoids found in cannabis because it does not produce any psychoactive effects on its own.

CBD may cause feelings of relaxation and sleepiness, but it will not create a high. That being said, quite a few CBD products also contain trace amounts of THC (less than

.03%); these products create more of a psychoactive high. Most CBD gummies do not contain any THC.

Although some CBD oil is synthetically produced, most CBD products are derived from hemp plants. Historically, legal restrictions have limited the production, sale, and consumption of hemp-based products. However, passage of the 2018 Farm Bill led to the federal decriminalization of these activities. As a result, non-THC CBD oil products derived from hemp are legal to sell, buy, and use/consume anywhere in the U.S. In states where recreational cannabis is legal, CBD products containing THC are also legal. Other state laws vary considerably by location. For the purposes of this guide, we focus on CBD gummies that do not contain THC.

How Do Gummies Differ from Other CBD Products

Gummies offer a unique experience for CBD consumers that sets them apart from tinctures, topicals, and other forms of CBD. Common properties of CBD gummies include the following:

Edible: Because gummies are consumed orally, they like other CBD edibles typically produce longer-lasting effects than other forms of CBD oil, such as tinctures or vape oils. However, the level of effects also depends on the gummy's CBD concentration.

Concentration: A CBD gummy may have a concentration of up to 100mg, but most have concentrations of 30mg per capsule or lower. The ideal CBD concentration depends on the consumer's body weight and CBD tolerance, as well as the amount of pain relief they desire. For most people who weigh less than 200 pounds and have moderate to severe pain, a 30mg CBD serving is sufficient. Those who weigh more than 200 pounds may prefer to take higher concentrations.

Isolate vs. full spectrum: Whether a CBD oil is considered isolate or full-spectrum depends on how the oil is formulated. Isolate CBD oils only contain THC, while full-spectrum oils retain the CBD along with other non-psychoactive cannabinoids like cannabicyclol (CBL) and cannabinol (CBN), essential oils known as terpenes, and other nutrients. Most CBD gummies sold today are full-spectrum because they produce more well-rounded feelings of relaxation and pain relief, which make them popular with consumers. However, some gummies are made from CBD isolate.

Flavor: CBD gummies come in a wide range of flavors, including fruity and herbal options. CBD has a naturally strong taste that some people dislike, and some flavored gummies mask the taste of CBD very well.

Sugar content: Some CBD gummies contain sugar, which makes them unsuitable for consumers with certain medical conditions (such as diabetes). However, most gummies have a fairly low sugar content. Additionally, most gummies contain at least 10mg of CBD and consumers will not eat more than three to four per dose. For those seeking sugar-free CBD gummies, plenty of options are available, as well.

Gluten-free/vegan: CBD consumers who are vegan or unable to eat gluten products can choose from a wide selection of gluten-free, vegan gummies. However, some gummies do not meet either/both of these criteria. For this reason, customers with these restrictions should carefully read the product label and reach out to company representatives if necessary.

Price: Price-points for CBD gummies vary by brand and individual product, but most are available for 20 cents per mg or less; this puts gummies on par with other CBD oil products in terms of overall cost. Keep in mind that 'per mg' refers to the total CBD concentration found in the container, and not the number of gummies. For instance, let's say a container of 30 5mg gummies is priced at $20. This puts the container at roughly 13 cents per mg, and roughly 67 cents per gummy.

Are CBD Gummies Safe

CBD gummies and most other products containing CBD oil are considered generally safe. Their relaxing and pain-relieving qualities are well documented, and side effects are minor (if not non-existent) for most consumers. However, CBD may lead to the following bodily issues:

- Dry mouth: Dry mouth is associated with most CBD products; cannabinoids may interact with receptors that control salivation, resulting in mild but uncomfortable dryness inside the mouth. Strong feelings of thirst may also occur. Gummies with high concentrations of fruit juice may limit dry mouth to some extent, but most CBD consumers find that drinking at least one glass of water will effectively curb dry mouth symptoms.

- Lower blood pressure: Some consumers experience a temporary drop in blood pressure immediately after taking CBD oil products. While this is not a serious issue for most, people with low blood pressure or those taking certain medications should check with their doctor before trying CBD products.

- Diarrhea: Large doses may upset the stomach and lead to digestive problems like diarrhea. Lower does are less likely to cause these problems.

- Changes in appetite: Increased appetite is a common side effect of CBD gummies, and CBD oil/cannabinoids in general. Because gummies are consumed as edible capsules, eating them may reduce hungry feelings to some extent.

Additionally, CBD gummies that contain sugar may not be suitable for people with diabetes or other conditions that restrict sugar intake. For these individuals, sugar-free gummies are the best option. As a rule, anyone who is interested in taking CBD products should always check with their doctor first. Low doses are recommended for first-time consumers.

Do CBD Gummies Get You High

CBD gummies produce feelings of relaxation in consumers; they also alleviate pains and other discomforts stemming from symptoms of different medical conditions. However, non-THC CBD gummies will not make consumers feel high in the same way that marijuana and other products with THC will. This is because CBD does not produce psychoactive effects like THC does.

Some but not all full-spectrum gummies with contain trace amounts of THC; in most cases, these products contain 0.3% of THC or less. They may cause extremely slight psychoactive effects but will not produce the same high as, say, edibles containing marijuana (which can be as much as 30% THC or higher).

And although CBD gummies may not produce a psychoactive high, they often cause consumers to feel sleepy. As a result, we advise consumers not to take CBD gummies if they plan to work with machinery, operate a motor vehicle, or engage in other activities that require full motor skills.

How to Eat CBD Gummies Responsibly

A CBD gummy may contain anywhere from 1mg to 100mg of CBD. However, most gummies sold today contain between 5mg and 30mg.

As we've noted, the optimal dosage for any given consumer will depend on his/her weight, tolerance to CBD, and desired effects. The table below lists general CBD concentration ranges for people based on their weight. However, we urge all first-time CBD consumers to begin with a relatively small dose (10mg or less) and then gradually increase the dosage until the desired effects are reached; this will likely create a more pleasurable experience than beginning with a high dose.

10 CBD Gummies

One of the most convenient and fun ways to take cannabidiol (CBD) is through CBD gummies. They're easy to dose (no measuring or droppers necessary), portable, discreet, and tasty, making them a good choice for people looking to try CBD for the first time. They may be helpful for various purposes, like quelling anxiety and helping with insomnia. It's important to know that not every gummy is created equal, however.

Since there are currently no over-the-counter (OTC) CBD products approved by the Food and Drug Administration (FDA), it's important to do your research and make sure you're buying a quality product.

Excited to dive in but don't know where to start? Here are 10 great options that have been closely evaluated in terms of their potency, CBD quality, and overall ingredients.

All of the products listed here are lab-tested, made from U.S.-grown cannabis, and have less than 0.3 percent tetrahydrocannabinol (THC).

Products

CBD GLOSSARY

You'll see the following terms mentioned in the products below. Here's what they mean:

- CBD isolate: pure CBD, with no other cannabinoids or THC
- Broad-spectrum CBD: contains most cannabinoids, but it generally doesn't include THC

- Full-spectrum CBD: contains all of the plant's cannabinoids, including THC

1. Lord Jones Old-Fashioned CBD Gumdrops

Lord Jones' CBD gumdrops are handmade in small batches with broad-spectrum CBD extract and natural fruit flavors. Each gluten-free gumdrop contains a generous 20 milligrams (mg) of CBD. With only nine gummies in a package, these are a little pricey, but let's be honest: These stylishly packaged gumdrops would make a great gift for a friend or even yourself. These contain zero THC, so they're a good option for those looking to avoid its effects entirely.

2. Sunday Scaries CBD Gummies

Sunday Scaries makes two types of gummies: gelatin-based, and pectin-based for vegans. Both versions are made from full-spectrum CBD and contain vitamins B-12 and D-3 which are especially great for vegans, who may not get enough of these vitamins in their diets.

While the vegan version contains high fructose corn syrup, the non-vegan version uses pure cane sugar instead. Both versions contain 10 mg of CBD per gummy and have 20 gummies in a bottle.

3. CBDfx Gummies with Turmeric and Spirulina

CBDfx's gummies contain turmeric, an anti-inflammatory, as well as spirulina, a superfood and antioxidant. Add some organic, broad-spectrum CBD into the mix and you wind up with a gummy that has rave reviews. They're vegan, GMO-free, and don't contain any artificial sweeteners or high fructose corn syrup.

Each bottle contains 60 gummies with 5 mg of CBD each. This is about the lowest dose you can get in a CBD product, so they're a good choice for beginners or people who don't need something highly concentrated.

4. Charlotte's Web CBD Gummies

Charlotte's Web CBD products first gained attention after being used for epilepsy, and they've remained a popular brand ever since. They offer a few types of CBD gummies, including Recovery, Sleep, and Calm blends.

The Recovery blend is geared toward those seeking additional anti-inflammatory properties, thanks to the addition of ginger and turmeric.

The Sleep blend is a good choice for those dealing with insomnia, since it has the added benefit of melatonin. The Calm blend has lemon balm and L-theanine to help with stress and anxiety. All gummies contain 10 mg of full-spectrum CBD, and there are 60 per package.

5. Highland Pharms CBD Gummies

These gummies are beloved by consumers for their great taste. Each 20-piece jar contains several flavors, and they come in 10 mg or 20 mg of CBD per gummy options. The CBD used is full-spectrum, and the gummies are made with all-natural flavors and colors, as well as some organic ingredients. They're gluten-free, but they're processed in a facility that handles soy and fish gelatin, so those with fish or soy allergies may want to choose a different gummy.

6. PlusCBD Oil Gummies

Another full-spectrum product, PlusCBD's vegan gummies are available in two flavors: cherry mango and citrus punch. And they're made without any artificial ingredients. They're also non-GMO, gluten-free, and soy-free, so they're a good choice for people with allergies. Available in 30-count or 60-count packages, they have just 5 mg of CBD per gummy great for those looking for a low-dose product.

7. Fab CBD Chews

These gummies are made with CBD isolate, making them a good option for people who want to avoid THC altogether. They're also vegan, non-GMO, and use natural colors and flavors. There are 30 gummies in a package, with 25 mg of CBD per gummy. This brand might not be a great choice for those with allergies, since its gummies are processed in a facility that handles soy and fish gelatin.

They're also packaged in a facility that handles wheat, peanuts, tree nuts including coconut, pistachios, and cashews as well as soy and milk products.

8. Hemp Bombs CBD Sleep Gummies

Tossing and turning all night. Say goodbye to counting sheep with Hemp Bombs' sleep gummies. The price is a little high on these, but there are 60 to a package.

Each gummy has 15 mg of organic, broad-spectrum CBD and 5 mg of melatonin. They also contain a blend of L-theanine, Scutellaria, and Passiflora, which may help with relaxation. These gummies use corn syrup as the sweetener. They also contain gelatin, so they aren't a good choice for vegans or vegetarians.

9. Joy Organics CBD Gummies

Made with only eight ingredients, Joy Organics use organic apple juice to flavor their gummies, and organic agave and stevia to sweeten them. Each gummy contains 20 mg of broad-spectrum CBD, and there are 15 gummies to a jar. They're THC-free, gluten-free, and vegan.

10. Pure Relief Pure Hemp Gummies

At 30 mg of CBD per gummy bear, these are some of the most potent CBD products out there. They offer two 30-count options: a daytime formula, and a nightime formula, which has the addition of melatonin. These contain CBD isolate, so they're a great option for consumers who may need higher doses of CBD but don't want to consume any THC.

How to choose
Use the following criteria when buying CBD gummies:

CBD source
The first thing to consider when purchasing CBD gummies is the type of CBD used. CBD isolate is pure CBD, with no other cannabinoids. While isolates are ideal for consumers who want to avoid THC, this extraction method strips away cannabis's volatile organic compounds and terpenes. This means the end result won't provide the full range of health benefits.

Products made with broad-spectrum CBD contain most cannabinoids, but generally don't contain THC. Products made with full-spectrum CBD contain all of the plant's cannabinoids, including THC. Full-spectrum products provide the most therapeutic benefits as a result of as the entourage effect, which means that cannabinoids have a greater effect combined than consumed alone.

The best bet is to go for a full- or broad-spectrum product made with organic hemp grown in the United States. Hemp grown in the United States is subject to agricultural regulations, and it can't contain more than 0.3 percent THC.

Any product that doesn't specifically say what type of CBD was used for instance, listing only "cannabis extract" as an ingredient is probably one to avoid.

Potency

Dose varies widely across CBD products, and it may depend on the CBD source. For example, a 5 mg full-spectrum CBD gummy may feel a lot more potent than a 5 mg CBD isolate gummy.

If you're unsure what dose to look for, the best bet is to start with the lowest one available — generally 5 mg and increase from there.

Ingredients

There's a lot more to CBD gummies than just CBD. Other ingredients can vary widely. Pay attention to additives like artificial ingredients and preservatives.

You may also want to avoid high fructose corn syrup, and if you're vegan or have allergies, look for products that match those needs.

The ideal CBD gummy is made with organic, non-GMO ingredients, real sugar, and natural flavorings. You can even purchase CBD products that contain vitamins or adaptogenic herbs.

Common additions include turmeric and spirulina, two nutrient-rich superfoods that have a wide range of health benefits.

Third-party testing

Since there are no OTC CBD products approved by the FDA, quality varies. Look for companies that test their products in a lab, preferably by a third party. Test results will tell you whether the product contains what it says it does. What to consider while shopping

- CBD source
- potency
- ingredients
- third-party testing

How to use

Most gummies come in packs of 20 to 60, and they're dosed at 5 mg or more of CBD per gummy. If you've never experimented with CBD, start with a 5 mg gummy. Some gummies can be cut in half so you can start with 2.5 mg.

Wait up to 2 hours to experience the full effects, and if you feel like you need more, experiment until you find your "just right" dose. You can consume gummies daily, but keep in mind the effects from a gummy tend to last 4 to 6 hours. Store in a cool, dark place away from sunlight.

Safety tips and side effects

CBD is non-intoxicating, meaning it won't get you high. It's generally recognized as safe, and there are few side effects, though they do occur occasionally.

- Possible side effects
- fatigue
- diarrhea
- changes in appetite
- changes in weight

Some research suggests that CBD may interact with liver enzymes and temporarily stop the liver from metabolizing other medications or breaking down toxins. Always consult your doctor before using CBD products.

HOW TO FIGURE OUT WHAT'S RIGHT FOR YOU

Experts recommend starting with a low dose 20 to 40 milligrams daily, according to Healthline's Medical Network (HMN) — and slowly increasing dosage over time until you find your "sweet spot."

Some folks find that taking a daily dose can help sustain a level of CBD in your body, which might stimulate your endocannabinoid system (more on what this is, below) to make it react more to cannabinoids like CBD.

And many people use a microdosing technique to find their personal dosage and adjust it as needed over time.

You may find it helpful to use a journal to log your results. Keep track of how much you've taken, how you feel before dosing and at several time intervals afterward, and any changes in symptoms that you notice.

Over time, this info can help paint a picture of how CBD affects you.

Keep in mind that it's possible to build up a tolerance to CBD, like many other drugs and chemicals. So if you find that it's not working as well after a while, try taking a few days' break to reset your system before starting with a low dose again.

YOU NEED TO GIVE IT MORE TIME

The first time I tried CBD, I wondered if I'd wasted my money on some overhyped trend. I put some drops of an oil tincture under my tongue, expected near-instant relief from my chronic pain, and got… nothing.

My experience isn't at all unusual, because immediate results aren't all that common.

In fact, many people take CBD for several weeks or even several months before they see a difference.

Exploring the effects of CBD isn't as simple as taking a couple of Tylenol and calling it a day. It actually requires a certain level of commitment to put time and thought into your process of uncovering the long-term effects.

If you're still not seeing results after a while (think a few months), then it may be time to move on and try a different brand. Your CBD journal can help you keep track of how long it's been and whether or not you've experienced any changes.Patience is key, and while it can be frustrating to keep trying with no results, you may end up feeling super grateful that you didn't give up.

YOU NEED A DIFFERENT DELIVERY SYSTEM

We're well aware that the CBD market is full of fly-by-night businesses that simply want to capitalize on the rapidly growing industry. The general lack of public awareness when it comes to testing the quality of Cannabidiol-infused goods is an industry-wide problem.

It seems like I'm hearing about a new CBD product just about every week. You can find everything from CBD coffee to bath salts and lube.

Common forms of CBD

- tinctures
- topical creams
- vape oils
- capsules or suppositories
- edible treats like gummies and chocolate

So if you've been trying one delivery system with no luck, it's possible that a different form would work better for you.

One factor to consider is bioavailability, which essentially refers to how much of the CBD actually gets into your bloodstream.

For example, if you eat CBD gummies, they have to go through your digestive tract before you can absorb them, and the amount that ends up in your system may be relatively low.

On the other hand, if you take a tincture sublingually — which means under the tongue — you're absorbing it directly into your bloodstream. So you could get quicker, more noticeable results than you would from waiting for your digestive system to process it.

In addition, your most effective method may vary depending on what type of relief you're looking for.

For example, a topical balm won't help you with your panic attacks. But it can offer potential relief for, say, sore muscles, if you zero in on that particular area.

CBD may be popular, but that doesn't mean it's a miracle drug that will work for everyone. After all of your efforts, it's possible that you'll find that CBD simply doesn't work for you.

YOUR LEVEL OF ABSORPTION AND REACTION TO CBD DEPENDS ON A VARIETY OF FACTORS INCLUDING YOUR:

- metabolism
- biochemistry
- genetics

Your endocannabinoid system is the system in your body that interacts with the active compounds in cannabis, and each person's operates a little differently.

In fact, a professor of clinical psychiatry noted 20 percent of Americans may have a genetic mutationTrusted Source that makes them naturally produce more endocannabinoids — similar to cannabinoids but produced by your body.

If you have that mutation, you might be prone to lower levels of anxiety, but because you already have extra endocannabinoids you might not see much of a difference when you take CBD.

CHECK WITH YOUR DOCTOR ABOUT OTHER OPTIONS THAT MAY WORK FOR YOU.

And if you have persistent friends, don't be afraid to tell them to stop bugging you about giving CBD a try. After all, there's no such thing as a one-size-fits-all treatment!

GETTING CBD TO WORK TAKES TIME, PATIENCE, AND RESEARCH

CBD isn't as well-researched or regulated as many other treatment options like prescription medications, and people within the industry are still trying to narrow down the best practices for taking it.

But one thing's for sure: It's not as simple as taking some standard dosage and seeing immediate results. It takes time, patience, and ongoing research to find the right brand, dosage, and delivery method for you.

Which means the process can also get pricey — as you might have to buy products from several different companies over the course of several months before you find what works.

Before you go all-in on a full-sized product from a reputable company that may cost a lot of money but might not work for you, check to see if you can buy sample packs of the product.

So before you give up on CBD altogether, use the above reasons as a check list to figure out why CBD isn't working for you.

Conclusion

CBD Gummies make for a fun and easy way to get the CBD you need. All you need to do is enjoy snacking on some tasty CBD treats to get the beneficial medical effects. What's more, they're split into easy-to-consume serving sizes to get the ideal dosage.

The dosage you need will depend on a lot of factors, although research now tells us which dosages are likely to work. There's also no harm in experimenting- if you find your dosage isn't working, you can safely increase it without negative effects. Bear in mind that, in some cases, you may need to give CBD a few weeks to build up in the body and have a more prominent effect.

CPSIA information can be obtained
at www.ICGtesting.com
Printed in the USA
FSHW020511110121
77568FS

9 781702 481984